How to Love a Woman Through Cancer

G. A. Robinson

authorHOUSE®

AuthorHouse™
1663 Liberty Drive
Bloomington, IN 47403
www.authorhouse.com
Phone: 1 (800) 839-8640

Published by AuthorHouse 01/20/2016

ISBN: 978-1-5049-7522-3 (sc)
ISBN: 978-1-5049-7521-6 (e)

Library of Congress Control Number: 2016901126

Print information available on the last page.

This book is dedicated to Connie Ann Baker, my love, my friend, my mother. Thank you. Peace, Love and Blessings. Namaste!

Some say cancer is a disease of dis-ease

Others say cancer is caused by cell confusion and molecular exclusions

But no matter what the reason we all have a season of cancer in our lives

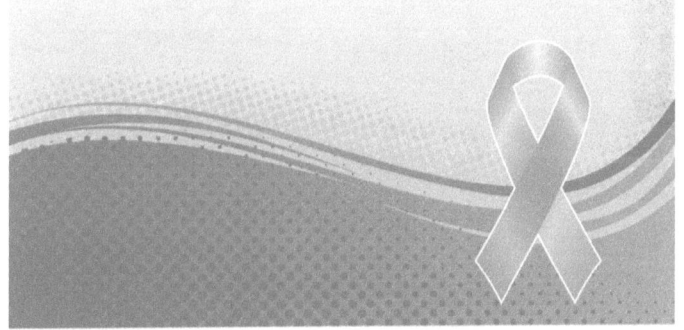

Sometimes its cancerous people

Sometimes its cancerous things

G. A. ROBINSON

Sometimes its cancerous tumors

Sometimes its cancerous days

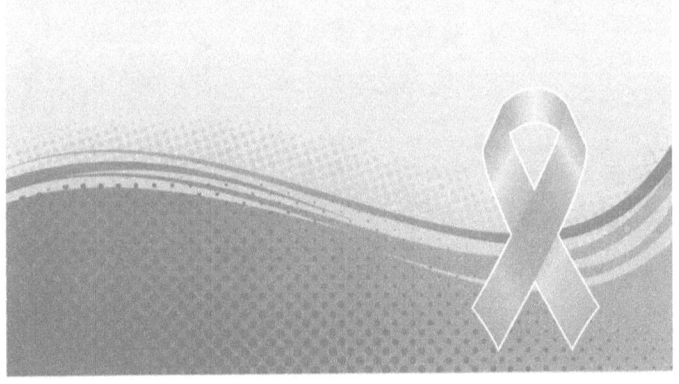

No matter what the reason for the cancerous season

It's important to love a woman through it and help her get to the other side

How do you love a woman through cancer?

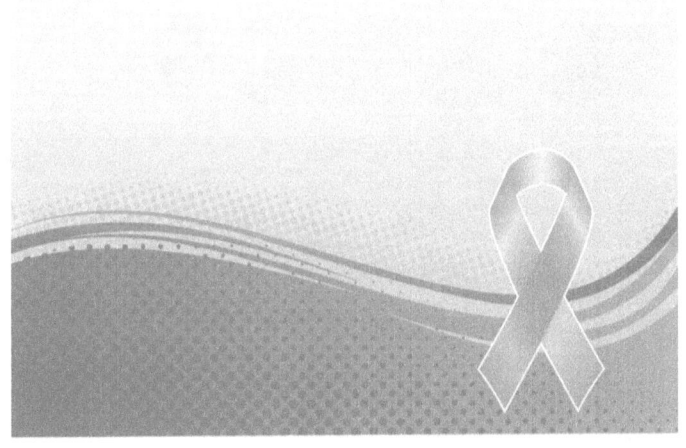

Well there are lots of ways

You can give her something shiny

Or something sweet

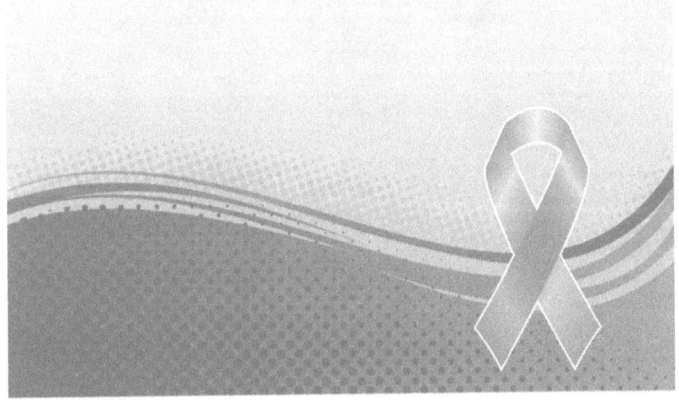

Give her things she been longing for

Or something to help her sleep

Give her something to make her smile

Or something healthy for her belly

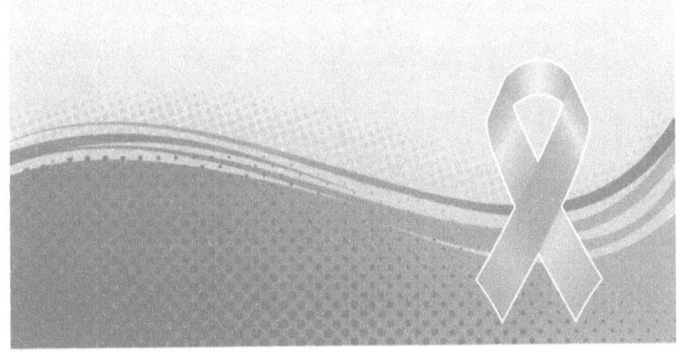

Give her a coloring book

Give her a second look

Give her a candle

Give her a purse with a pretty handle

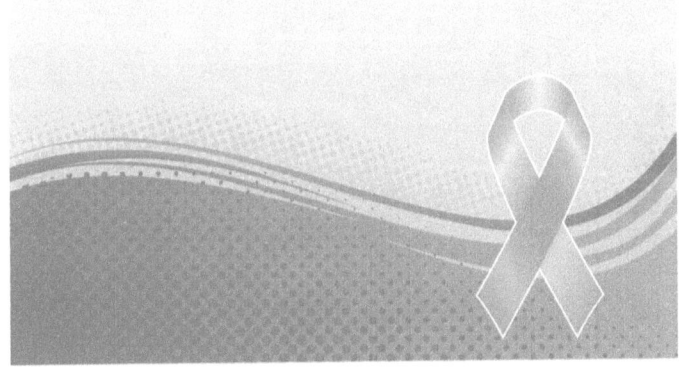

Give her a wig

Give her a plant

Give her a nice paperweight

Give her a t-shirt

Give her a bracelet

Take her for a haircut

Take her for a ride around the world or just around town

Sit with her at chemo

Hold her hand at radiation

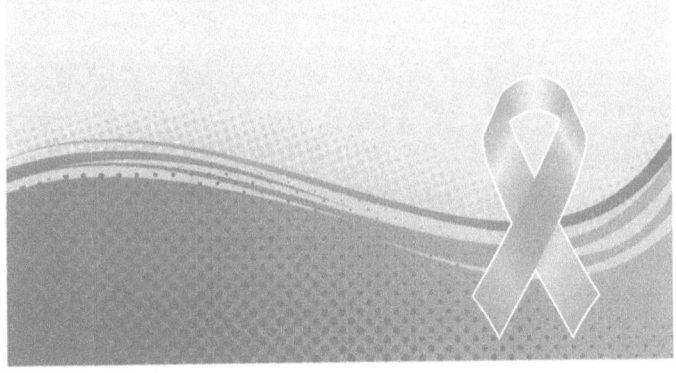

Make sure she has saltines when her tummy hurts

Read her a poem

Share a meal

Share a drink

Listen to her story

Tell her what you think

Give her a book or a kindle now a days

Let her Cry, tear up, Cry some more then scream and don't leave

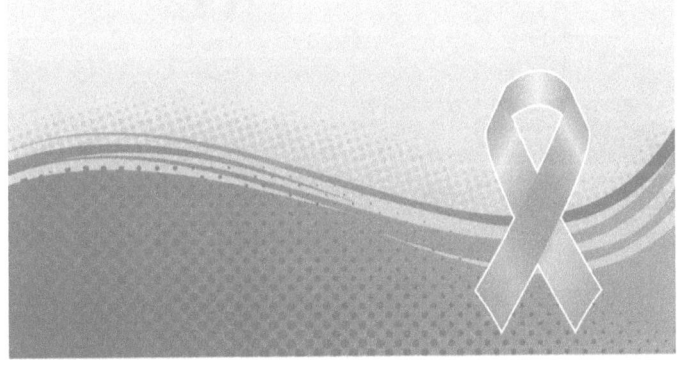

Tell her it will be ok

Let her learn to love herself in a new and very special way

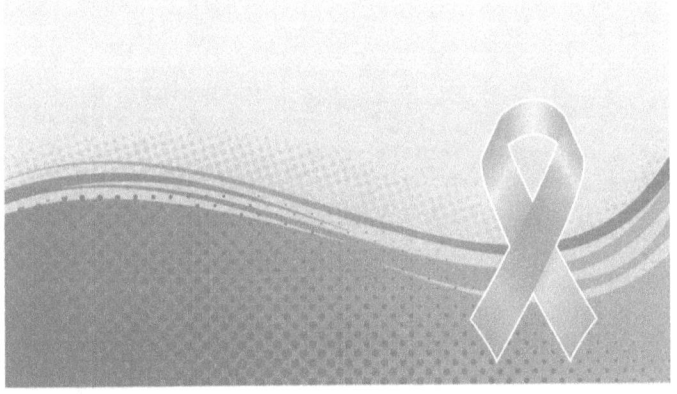

Help her see her beauty

Help her move past the past

Say it will be ok (even if you don't know)

Say this too shall pass (even if it may not be the end you prefer)

Focus on the future

Reminisce

Draw her a picture

Tell her a joke

Take her to a play or movie

Exercise with her

Take her to a sporting event

Put on her favorite TV show

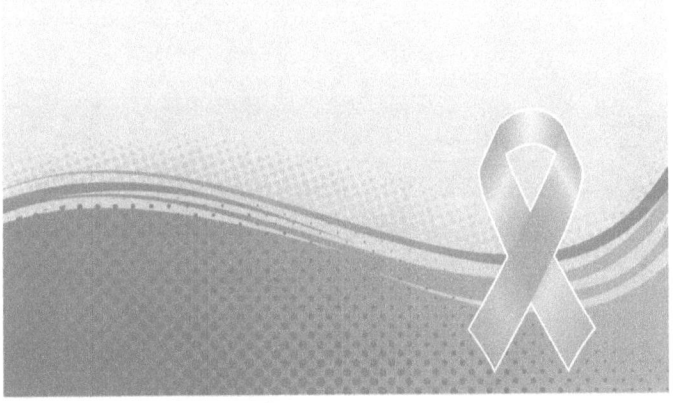

Hide her when she doesn't want to be seen

Tell her how much you love her

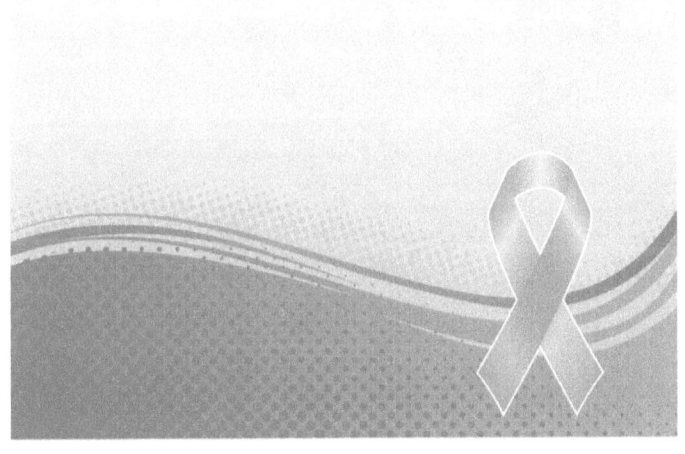

Sing her favorite song

Write her a love song

Help her Break the rules (ice cream before dinner)

Help her write a list of people she will forgive

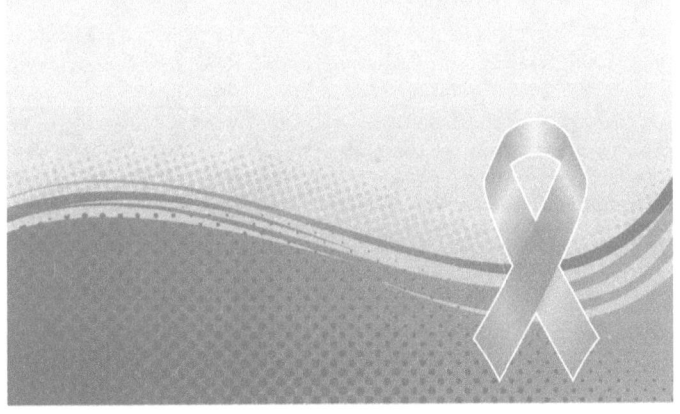

Clean her house

Pay a bill

Take her on a trip

Give her a thrill

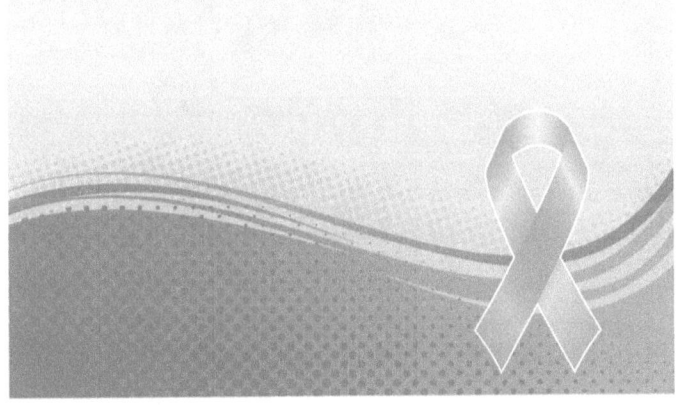

Give her a massage

Mediate/Pray/Find something to believe in together

Or not

Laugh at each other

Help her plan on how she will give more

Share new dreams

Reinvent your relationship together and evolve into your newness

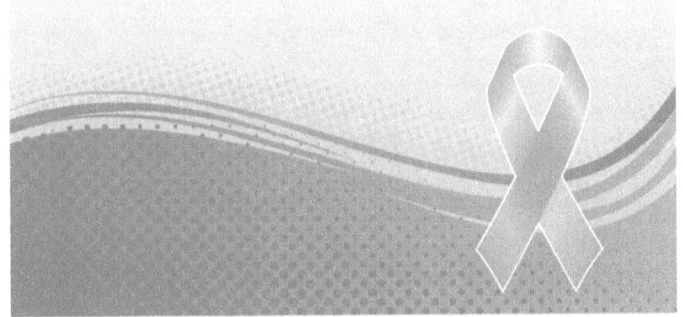

Give her, her favorite perfume

Give her a blanket

Give her a robe

Give her a balloon bouquet

Paint her nails

Make her Tea

G. A. ROBINSON

Fix her favorite meal

Wash the dishes

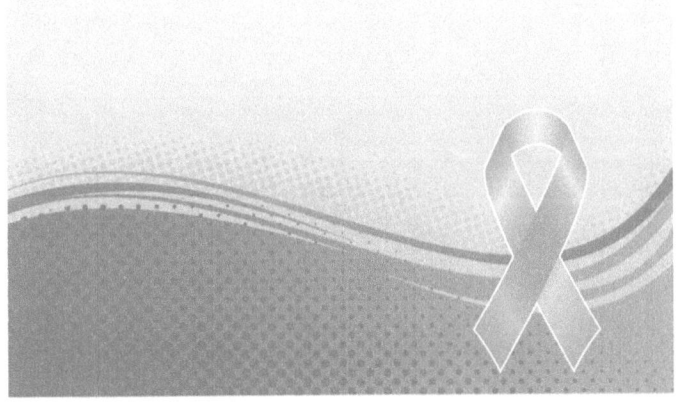

Finish her to-do list

Watch her favorite movie with her

Dress up for no reason at all

Dress down and wear a hat

Wear PJs with feet and slide across the floor right into her lap

Take her for a dip in the pool (if the doctors say ok)

Listen to music 2 gether

Make some music for each other

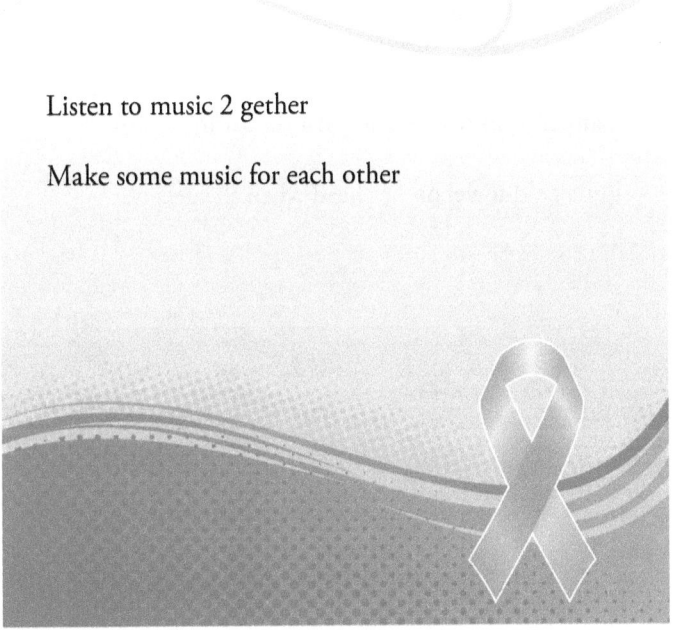

Turn the air on high then turn it off and give her a blanket (until its time to turn the air up again)

Put a cold towel on her head when she gets hot

Make her a bubble bath

Give her a big hug

Make her a sandwich

Light a smell good candle

Tell her nice things

Go to a park together and swing

Get a dog or a cat

Show her love in your own very special way

Kiss her

Believe in her and just love her.